Powerful Modern Motivating Quotes to Fuel Your Exercise and Wellness

Boost Your Physical and Mental Toughness Effortlessly

SAMSON YUNG-ABU

PublishNation
www.publishnation.co.uk

The author has an undergraduate degree in law & criminology, a postgraduate degree in general law, a law school in Berlin certificate, and a MSc degree in psychology. The author is a life-long creator turned tutor who enjoys motivating people across the world, teaching and inspiring others about the joys of life and education.

Intro

The mountain won't climb itself; it won't physically pull you up to its summit. However, its imposing height and intimidating presence can inspire you to want to conquer it. Through its quiet existence and powerful presence, it inspires you to say, "You do not surpass my courage to overcome you, and I will demonstrate that immediately!" This is the strength of motivation; it renders everything conquerable. Your fitness and well-being represent this mountain. Your health and wellness symbolise this mountain. The question at this point is, is your mountain more powerful than you? Does its height exceed your bravery? And the key question is this: Are you able to overcome it? If so, demonstrate it—to yourself and for your well-being.

R egardless of whether you visit the gym or choose to exercise at home, having motivation can determine whether you abandon your fitness goals or accomplish them consistently. To enhance your motivation, this book is ideal to support you while exercising.

No matter who you are, sometimes you just don't feel energised or motivated somedays to do what you frequently do with ease. On days like this, a pick-me-up motivational quote can go a long way to replenish your energy and help you feel fuelled enough to show up and put in the hard work required to build and impressive fitness and wellness.

From celebrated sports figures to distinguished writers and leading figures globally, motivation serves as a vital resource that fuels their drive and inspires them to persevere and overcome challenges! Even if you don't require it at the moment, keep it prepared. Get ready for your days of mental gloom.

A note to take with you on your fitness journey is this: reaching our fitness goal can be a tug of war between what we want on one hand and, on the other hand, what is keeping us from achieving our desires: distractions, tempting high-calorie foods, hectic schedules, inadequate diet plans, family obligations, cozy couches, low energy, self-doubt, mental health struggles, and so on. The inspiring quotes in this book are the phrases that have motivated me to persist through my individual, social, and economical challenges. These phrases have helped me navigate the challenging phases of my fitness journey. What we need to realize is that reaching your goal will not be simple. Nevertheless, there exists a system that aids us in managing the most challenging parts of the process, allowing us to move forward effectively until we arrive at our intended goal. You don't need to constantly pressure yourself every single day. You can also move yourself ahead effortlessly. This is what motivational quotes can achieve for us: Ease.

Why are motivational quotes important in fitness? Motivational quotes in fitness are essential since the path to fitness can be mentally challenging, and we need inspiration to bolster our minds while we aim for our ideal bodies and holistic health. Achieving fitness success follows a system that includes dieting, exercising, and engaging in other pertinent healthy activities to reach a desired result. This system also depends on our comprehension of what actions to take, awareness of how to execute them properly, actually doing it and the aspect that many of us find challenging: the desire to do it at all. This is where inspirational quotes become relevant..

What do motivational quotes signify in fitness? To me, motivational quotes are comprehensive success advice compressed into a few words for easy reading and application. In general, I believe that motivational quotes have a similar effect to those long, adaptable breathing tubes filled with air to boost athletes' stamina; what they do to you in fitness is encourage you to exceed your mental and physical boundaries when you are fed up, tired, out of breath, and nearing your limits. Yet, based on individual interpretation, they can signify different meanings; however, regarding fitness, and for this book's context, in one word, motivational quotes also represent footprints. Why footprints? As defined by the Oxford Dictionary, a footprint signifies "the mark made by a foot or shoe on the ground or a surface." In fitness motivational quotes are footprints because they represent guidance and direction toward a goal embraced by those who achieved that objective. When we analyse it rationally, even from a scientific standpoint, motivational quotes offer a framework for achievement while also detailing actions to pursue and those to evade during the whole journey, ultimately, they provide confirmations, instructions and directions when action to a specific destination is intented.

The truth is that each motivational quote stems from a journey that involved key elements like dedication, persistence, self-discipline, commitment, pride, resolve, setbacks, and, in the end, achievement. The presence of these footprints drives us to continue on. They motivate us to confidently follow the routes already laid out through the direction, teachings, advice, and restrictions integrated into our mindset.

In addition, one lesson I discovered on my fitness journey is that mental readiness is a crucial asset to possess, and neglecting to prepare is essentially consenting with failure to do its worst, run its course, and get away with damage.

As a person who originally encountered more setbacks than successes in my fitness journey, I soon recognised the beneficial influence of following daily motivational messages. This book, hence, includes impactful words and ideas that have maintained my discipline, motivation, commitment, consistency, and focus in my journey to achieve fitness, health, and happiness. I am confident you will find them influential as you strive to become the healthiest version of yourself. As you browse this amazing collection of quotes, I wish you the best of luck on your fitness journey.

Fitness isn't a journey you start afresh or decide to take up on January first. It's something you bring into every moment of your day and throughout the entire year.

If you want to burn anything down, you've got to first light the fire. The same goes for burning those excess calories. You can't burn them off by sitting around waiting or complaining. You've got to ignite the fire, and your working out is the fire.

In pursuing our fitness goals, it's less about what we have or don't have that can benefit our health and more about our attitude. The physical elements of achieving fitness success account for only 30%. Seventy percent of the hard work needed is based on our view of how valuable our time and effort are. Therefore, whether or not we possess physical resources like high-end fitness gear, a luxury workout space, or trendy athletic wear, until we have faith in ourselves and recognise our value, it will often appear unfeasible to start, achieve, or maintain any progress in fitness.

If you don't feel or look healthy, it's due to having set your self-care standards too low. You've allowed your health to decline as you've concentrated your time and energy on matters that have provided minimal benefit to your physical, mental, and emotional wellness. You must shift your attention, for without excellent health, nothing else accomplished will hold value for you.

As you pursue your fitness goals, if you find yourself in an environment that is full of criticism, do two things: (1) listen and (2) do not take it as a fact. Only what we accept as true is true, and the power to accept is always yours to express. One thing I also discovered is that criticism can be a source of emotional strength. Criticism can create a monstrous mind capable of conquering everything in sight. So listen and let it motivate you to work harder to prove everyone wrong about their doubts regarding your ability to excel in your fitness journey.

.

Achieving positive health isn't just about doing what we prefer, but about enduring what we hate until we fall in love with it, which is bound to happen. Without sugarcoating it, the process may be monotonous and laborious. Nonetheless, it took me some time to get through the repetitive nature of workouts and meal plans. What helped me was understanding that I preferred to be bored and healthy, joyful and stronger, rather than entertained but miserable, unhealthy, and unhappy. Currently, I enjoy engaging in all the aspects that I previously hated.

Everything great starts with guts and grit. You won't encounter growth until you've dug deep. And that takes instant and continuous action. What we must also understand is that not doing your best is at your emotional, physical, and social expense. The cost arrives with sorrow, with suffering, with lost of time, and with overlooked chances. Similar to other aspects of my life where I have found success, I understood that to enhance my health, I must challenge myself mentally, emotionally, and physically everyday to accomplish my goals. If not, no one will motivate me, assist, or drive me, and I will be the sole person experiencing what follows.

One major key ingredient to fitness improvement is movement. Fitness doesn't have to be all pressure and torture; it can also be pleasure through doing something fun and exciting. At times, all you require is your headphones on, upbeat music blasting, and you dance until your legs are sore, your blood surges wildly through your veins, and your body feels like you've just completed a 100-meter dash. Whatever movement gets your heart racing counts toward the improvement of your health.

You can't just half-ass your way to a positive health. You've got to be a badass, which means you have to show up even when it's tough, even when it's cold, raining, or too hot. You've got to push through even when you feel broken, even when the odds are against you. You've got to do what others won't do, especially in those tough moments when others might flee.

To attain success in your fitness journey, you must daily train your mind to reliably inspire itself to take the actions you desire before it leads you to make an unwelcome choice. Here is where individual discipline is crucial. It calls for a more impartial assessment of the pros and cons of the options at your disposal, being more aware and determined about how each choice will either aid or obstruct your fitness objectives.

At the beginning of my fitness journey, I struggled and failed. I made errors that caused me a few setbacks. But I wasn't ready to give up. I started again, and this time it was slow and steady. Today, I realised that it isn't about how badly you started; it's about how much you want to end up better. I am better because of my starting experience.

Don't wake up just to give up. Don't show up just to slow down. Don't start something just to quit it. Get up and level up! Fight that fear. Fight that doubt. Fight the odds. Fight that soothing voice that wants you to stay under the covers and chill out. If you want to become stronger, faster, healthier, and happier, you can't afford to skip a planned workout session or give in to quitting.

I frequently tell individuals wanting to shed pounds this: Your heart is your health scale. Quit depriving yourself of food merely to shed pounds and appear thin. Eat nutritious foods. Certainly, track your progress, but remember that a drop in the scale's numbers doesn't automatically indicate positive results: less weight doesn't always equal improvement. Has your level of stress gone down? Has your rest gotten better? Have you ceased negative thoughts? Has your self-worth improved? These are questions a scale can't provide feedback on. But your heart can. Therefore, exercise caution and refrain from evaluating your health solely based on the scale's figures. You are not a grocery item. You are not a fruit or vegetable. Your weight does not directly indicate your health. Your internal feelings on the other hand, offer precise insight into your improving health.

The thing with fitness is that the work is never done. It requires ongoing effort to uphold and keep. Just because you've made it this far doesn't mean you should cease your hard work to advance further. Taking a break is fine, but complacency sets in when we replace resting with settling.

Exercise caution when testing boundaries. Certainly, concentrate on progression, but also be mindful of your body's boundaries. Test yourself, but don't hurt yourself. Individuals who are more likely to maintain their exercise and diet routines realise that enhancing fitness isn't about quickness or intensity; it's about the consistency in how you allocate your time and energy toward both results and recovery. It's not about pushing yourself constantly, overexerting, and putting yourself at risk of injuries. With an injury, it will become harder to push harder or go further, anyway. Therefore, maintain a healthy speed, and the outcomes will undoubtedly be visible.

A key piece of advice that has kept me in a winning zone is recognising and accepting that there are specific elements of success I cannot delegate to luck or anyone else but myself. I am both the leader and the builder. In achieving success in your fitness journey, laziness is a decision. Choosing to be inactive is also a decision. These options are harmful to building. To build anything significant, you can't rely on luck, coincidence, or convenience. Whether heavy or rough, raining or cold, you've got to pick up the building blocks yourself and lay them one by one, day by day. In conclusion, what you desire won't occur for you unless you are prepared to be committed and engaged in the development process.

If you are just beginning to work on your health and still not seeing results. Be patient. Sometimes all you need is some more time invested in it. It will show soon enough as long as you don't quit.

Each year, if you prioritise comfort instead of your well-being, you'll end up in a worse condition than you are currently in. Your health won't simply remain stagnant while you unwind and pass the day putting things off. At this exact moment, your health is either getting better or worse, and the longer you let it decline, the harder it is to turn around. You can choose to do it voluntarily and with effort now, while it's easier and the physical demands are lower, or do it more intensely later when you're uncomfortable, feeling awful, and forced to exercise while having difficulty moving like you used to.

A diet plan, whether it is a low-carb or a low-fat diet, no matter how perfect it is, is only as effective as the mindset of the person using it. For instance, if you are a construction worker, the tools you have, no matter how technologically advanced or flashy they are, won't build the structure you want if you are too lazy to show up or tend to procrastinate on the job. Therefore, you need not just the expertise or the fancy tools but also the character to complete that job. The job, in this case, signifies your fitness goals.

If sticking to a diet or working out will change your life for the better, then make time for it, and work for it because you are worth it. The simple reality is that no one is ever too occupied to focus on their health. The issue for people who are overly busy isn't time; rather, it's a matter of value, particularly how much they prioritise their health compared to other aspects of life.

I view my fitness goals as my Goliath: large, but certainly conquerable. Those who succeed aren't succeeding merely because they aren't lazy. Everyone is battling something. Everyone is succeeding, and no one has it simple. What sets individuals apart is their willingness to face greater challenges. They are willing to take on a bigger opponent, one that those who see only small results aren't willing to confront. The truth is this: The magnitude of your victory is determined by the size of your opponent. If David hadn 't arrived with self-belief, no one would see his greatness, leaving Goliath as the major threat. If your health is your major threat, your Goliath, you can't play it small, you can't ignore it, you can't substitute it for smaller challenges and expect greater results. To defeat it, you must step forward and confront your Goliath to discover what you are made of and what you can become.

A lion that doesn't chase after living prey will soon struggle, or be incapable, of approaching a dead one. This is the outcome of neglecting our health. Good health will continuously elude us if we don't pursue it, if we don't strive for it! The more we permit it to slip away, the more vulnerable we are likely to grow.

I enjoy lifting weight because there is just something magical or mysterious about lifting heavy dumbbells or kettlebells and watching your body stretching, lengthening and strengthening. It kind of makes one feel instantly light, in a stressless sense: Like the worst things in your life fades with every weight exercise movement.

Someone once asked me why I prefer to work out at home rather than at the gym? There's nothing wrong with the gym, but here's why: One of the great things about working out at home is that you don't need to travel anywhere to transform your body. At home, you are always ready to get fit. At home, every room is a space. Every second is an opportunity. Any home wear is suitable for getting fit, and every movement can be done without feeling ashamed of being judged. There's just too much freedom when it comes to getting fit at home compared to anywhere else.

Many people regret each day not being able to stick to a specific diet plan. That's the problem: a single diet plan. If you are unable to stick to a diet plan, pick out another health-focused alternative that you can dedicate yourself to and observe the results. Enhancing fitness revolves around experimentation and error. It took me some time to discover what works best for me. What worked for me doesn't have to work for you. As long as you are trying, you will eventually find something that you can stick with.

Reaching your fitness goals won't be an overnight turnaround. You won't go to bed and awaken to immediately see the benefits or the loss of weight. You can't just rise and shine; you've got to rise and sweat before the shine comes!

You can't be upset about your weight issue while also feeling fine about not wanting to exercise and improve it. Play your role! Uncurl yourself, show up, check in, and begin making progress.

Never regret putting your health first. Respect it. Embrace it. Celebrate it. And do it repeatedly. You are surely worth it.

When God readies you for greatness, He frequently leads you through suffering, humiliation, remorse, and constraints. Since He understands that these are your keys to the destiny that He has already arranged for you. It's perfectly fine to be where you currently are; this is all a part of the journey toward your destined place: greatness! Just ensure that you do your part in the best way you can. Remember the words: "Heaven helps those who help themselves." Success is simply a matter of collaboration in action.

Real change occurs not when we desire something different but when we no longer want what we are currently experiencing. So sometimes, you've just got to look at change differently. You know. Rather than waking up wishing for things to change, just wake up and be done for a change: done with being unhappy and unhealthy. Done with feeling drained. Done with being overworked, underpaid, and unappreciated. Done with setting the bar too low and feeling like all you get are crumbs. Done with putting too much effort into things and receiving nothing in return. Sometimes you've got to be frustrated with your life before you can thrive in it. It's often how fed up you are with a situation that determines your next move for the rest of the year to change it.

What aids me in maintaining focus on my fitness journey is imagining that every day, starting from the moment I wake up, I am being televised, with my family, friends, and everyone globally observing my every action. I stay determined as I want to prevent disappointing myself, but also because I aim to maintain my efforts, understanding that many individuals may need a bit of encouragement for themselves that day. This awareness keeps me in check daily.

It's normal to feel anxious and afraid. It's natural to question if the downs will outweigh the ups when you begin focusing on bettering your health. Regardless of the situation, do not let your head get in the way of improving your body. Even if you doubt your ability to actually create your ideal body, put those uncertainties aside and think that you can. Put in your utmost effort. You had be surprised how much it's all in your head once you overcome your fear of starting and begin.

To achieve your preferred physique, you need to put your body through some discomfort and stress. At times, you must step out of the shadow of your comfort zone, spend more time on a not-so-comfortable weight bench instead of your cosy couch, and progressively lift weights that push you beyond comfort. Occasionally, you must move and run past your initial capability or painfully cut back on your favourite stress-relieving go-to snacks. Indeed, it may not be pleasant to express it this way, but that's the reality. That's how you improve your health; that's how you learn to cultivate it.

Days off are great. They are essential because they contribute to creating the ideal body you aspire to. However, for your days off to count, those days off must come after you've worked your ass off. Otherwise, there won't be any payoff.

It is up to you to press pause or play, but be wise enough not to half-ass it and smart enough not to go overboard. When you feel fatigued, take a break; and once you feel refreshed, make sure to get back to it immediately. Achieving a beneficial and valuable outcome depends on equilibrium rather than intensity.

You don't get anywhere great by being tired; you don't get anywhere great by being lazy. You don't get anywhere great through procrastination. You don't get anywhere great by wanting things to be easy. You get anywhere great by being determined, consistent, and passionate about winning. You've got to have that instinct to win at all costs within you.

Once you start saying yes to yourself instead of worrying about what others may or may not think of you, that is when you will stop living below your potential and begin to exceed judgments.

Do what makes your heart glow brightly. Let it feel like a sunny day wherever you go.

A friend of mine once mentioned that I desire to change, you see. However, I struggle to rise early in the morning no matter what, as I am not someone who enjoys mornings. Are you unable to or are you choosing not to? When we desire something intensely, we need to begin behaving like a different individual than we currently are. You cannot stay the same or act the same and anticipate a different result. Rise early; rise uniquely. That's the way to improve yourself beyond your current state. If rising early will enhance my intelligence, I will do it. If getting up early will improve my health, I will do it. If getting up will boost my energy, then I will.

Often, a positive change demands that we make some tough sacrifices by going to war with the version of ourselves that we currently are. So, take advantage of today's opportunity by not being afraid to challenge who you are in order to change. Step up, raise the bar, and rise to a new level of excellence.

I work hard on myself every day because I am too blessed to aim lower or settle for less than the best.

If you are willing to acknowledge that your health requires your focus and effort, it won't be an issue if you have insufficient money, time, or space for it. The reason for your lack of desire to do it won't be important. What's important is that you appear today, tomorrow, and the day following, and once you begin to do this, nothing will hinder you from accomplishing it. Does it really matter, or do your couch, TV, phone, bed, and friends take precedence over enhancing and safeguarding your well-being? The answer to your question is found in what you do next.

A lot of people are waiting for you to quit today. They are anticipating that you won't show up, as you said you would. They are ready to say, "What 's new? We knew it. Once a quitter, always a quitter." Do not give them that satisfaction today. Change the script. Change the narrative. Let them eat their words while you show up and demonstrate your worth and commitment. Today, be devoted to these words: no one is going to outshine me! No one is going to outperform me. No one is going to out-badass me. This is my competition. I will get up, get in that ring for my workout, and make a statement.

Each lesson learned unlocks a pathway to your greatest season so far. Therefore, continue to push your limits, keep acquiring knowledge, keep growing, and savour every moment because you've deserved it.

Looking back, what really impacted me this year were the chances I seized instead of letting them slip away. I seized every opportunity presented to me, and when there were none to be found, I made my own. Therefore, take advantage of any chance you encounter and make the most of it.

The best way to lose weight is to lose your unhealthy habits.

The period of comfort has passed; now is the time to show up and grow. Will it be easy? No. Will it be worth it? Absolutely yes. But first, you've got to show yourself some tough love to get through the hard times. Challenges aren't there to make us feel weak; they are there to help us discover just how strong we are when push comes to shove. Let's go.

Each day you rise to exercise, make certain that you progress solely at your own speed. Creating a better physique isn't for showing off; it's about enhancing yourself. Therefore, don't stress about the pace of others or how much ahead they are in their fitness progression. The only competition you need to focus on is the one between the you who wants to change and the you who doesn 't want to do what it takes. And that's the battle those who are further ahead wake up to fight and win day in and day out. So when you show up today, don't toy with your competition. Don't take your eyes off that fight. You didn't show up to impress anyone today but yourself. You didn't come to blend in or flaunt; you came to eradicate your health issues. That is your primary focus. Nothing else is relevant or required.

Sometimes, achieving your fitness goals and looking amazing in the end requires appearing odd, foolish, eccentric, or overly dedicated. Therefore, do not allow their criticism to hinder your growth. Success usually starts with the stares but always ends with the cheers. Keep going.

You are not supposed to control people's actions, only your own outcomes. That's what matters; that is what counts.

You could either wait for a lucky day or create the change you wish for yourself; however, to create that change, you must abandon your comfort zone, apply some pressure on yourself, push yourself a little harder than usual, and crush it.

If you want the gains you have to also have the pain. They are like a pair of shoe. And you can't walk around without the other.

Your first rep of the day is lifting yourself out of bed. But don't stop at that. You are stronger than just one rep.

I woke up today and had to choose between my weights or my worries again. I chose my weights. No matter how heavy they are, no matter how many weight plates I sensibly and safely add on, somehow they always feel lighter than my worries. Knowing that I can lift that much gives me hope that I can handle my worries too.

A lot of us are struggling to get fit and healthy because we are trying to stop our haters from hating on us when we try. But let them hate away; that's their job: to make noise, to judge you, and to demotivate you. Here is what you must do, though: stay focused on yourself. Your task isn't to prevent them from hating, but to quiet them, and that will only occur— not by you giving up or trying to satisfy them, but by you progressing and succeeding regardless.

Each workout provides me with a sense of relief because the visible sweat during exercise feels like my stress leaving my body. By the end of that session, I feel completely empowered and calm.

Whatever it is that you desire and want, don't wait until the universe gets around to you. Don't wait until coincidence comes knocking. Make it happen through your choice to want it. It is your birthright to receive it right away.

I don't turn every workout day into a day of physical advancement. There are days when I simply show up and workout to irritate the lethargic side of myself that prefers inaction. For me, being physically active at times is less about my physical state and more about my mentality. It's about developing and reinforcing the connection between my mentality and my drive to continue, no matter how I feel. This helps me develop the mental resilience needed to manage different aspects of my life.

For me these days, maintaining fitness and health seems like a cycle of inspiration. At times, I find motivation simply by observing myself: my reflection, my images, or videos documenting my health journey throughout the years, all of which remind me of the progress I've made in my well-being. It's an incredibly fulfilling sensation that motivate s me to continue. I am confident that there are people who feel this way, enduring and accomplishing more than they ever thought achievable. Therefore, commit to it and record every stage of your fitness process. It will carry more importance in the future as you continuously strive to enhance your health.

In this phase of my life, I am taking on the role of the challenger and no longer perceiving myself as an intruder regarding what I rightfully deserve. I will no longer seek permission. The goal now is to have the freedom to feel stronger, healthier, and more content. These are my priorities; they should take precedence over everything else.

When experiencing feelings of being overwhelmed or overloaded, the smartest choice isn't to indulge in comfort food but to exercise to dispel your cravings, uplift your mindset, and reduce your stress. When it's completed, you will feel significantly improved compared to earlier.

At times, I feel too exhausted to exercise, yet my stubbornness prevents me from yielding, so I still attend and get my workout done. When I complete it, I feel as though I have succeeded by not giving up.

Don't allow your body to endure pain tomorrow simply because you were too unwilling to exercise today. Of course, the decision is up to you. You can choose to have it simple now or improve it for tomorrow. Nonetheless, prior to making a selection, understand the distinction. The latter will require you to put in a lot of effort, but it will pay off for you in the end. The former, conversely, may need no effort at the moment, but it will lead to eventual pain and remorse.

One thing I can guarantee you is this: the more you train, the less you will have to complain. So if you want to win against your health problems, keep quiet for a little while and train hard.

Few statements carry as much truth as the phrase, "Health fosters happiness," and we can only genuinely appreciate life through good health. However, when the desire for making money eclipses the affection for nurturing, we lose sight of life's essence: happiness.

There is no rise without force. Therefore, cease desiring that things be simple or comfortable. Acknowledge that obstacles are essential and advantageous. When you confront them, they empower you and make you feel worthy, and the wonderful thing about it is that when everything is concluded, it demonstrates that you are more than you or others initially believed.

Learn to trust the process and believe that you are favoured, because God will not put you through the impossible. He may throw in what's unbearable and what can make you miserable, but it won't be anything unmanageable or unsolvable, because you are always going to be more than capable of achieving anything imaginable.

Triumph isn't solely about achieving a breakthrough; it's also about possessing a champion's mentality, which includes experiencing defeat and subsequently overcoming the challenges. The majority of individuals dislike obstacles; they favour a smooth journey without issues. However, setbacks are essential since experiencing failure and subsequently recovering is an important aspect of your development. The comeback after a setback is the flavour of your success; it is what makes the journey much sweeter in the end.

To succeed, you need to alter the "What if?" The "if" signifying "I'm fearful" to "I am capable of this!" Everything you long for isn't situated behind "what ifs"; it can solely be discovered ahead, past your "what ifs." We know that hard work pays off, so there's no need for you to stress about the results; trust that it is certain to occur eventually. So, what is it that scares you? The work involved? Trying to understand things? Staying dedicated to the fitness program even when it becomes challenging? Feeling fearful or unsure isn't about worrying if you'll accomplish your goals after exerting effort, but it is about not being ready to do what it takes.

As you begin to focus on your health and notice improvements, your outlook on life will start to shift, along with your priorities. You will become aware of decluttering your environment in a manner that will start to reward you with greater abundance in life.

A lesson I've discovered regarding fitness success is that obstacles are inevitable. There is always a considerable chance of getting hurt or valuing food more than your health routine after a time of doing the contrary. Simply recognising a loss doesn't imply that you've embraced defeat. You don't have to rush back into the ring to confront an opponent who appears more alluring or strong than you. Your opponent could, adhering to a diet, sticking to your workout regimen, or setting aside time to be with a partner or friend. Sometimes, following a setback, it's essential to go back to the drawing board rather than just getting back up and hoping to succeed right away.

Some people I knew or grew up with were comfortable being good and useful. I wasn't. I had to press the reset button on my destiny. I had to invest in being a beginner again, starting afresh and unafraid. So, if the path you are on seems like it isn't taking you anywhere, you don't have to keep going through it. Find the exit button and start a new path. What I finally understood was that sometimes you have to sacrifice the good to make room for the best things to come into your life.

I believe we often overlook the immense power each of us holds to bring our visions to life. I hadn't until I did, and that transformed everything for me. You're not obligated to live your life in a way that isn't true to you. You are not obligated to agree to conditions that make you uneasy. The power to alter any reality is a superhuman skill that every person has, including you. You simply need to turn it on and attain your goals with it.

I tell people all the time, don't just get the diet plan right; get your mindset right. A diet plan can only be effective with a strong mindset. You can't overlook your mindset and presume a strategy will succeed, even a carefully designed strategy. Diet plans written down are only as effective and impactful as the mindset that applies them. Consequently, your chances of achieving fitness success improve if you master the skill of discipline.

Today is a present. Avoid misusing it. Don't squander it. Do not underestimate it. Don't sell it for anything below its value. Instead, engage in actions that will enhance the value of your life.

If you want to accomplish and maintain positive health, you must stop spending all your energy thinking about the physical part of what you have to do and start considering why it matters that you get up frequently and do it without fail. You cannot underestimate the mental component of progress and anticipate achieving success in it.

Reaching your goal will not be easy, but it will definitely be rewarding. The obstacles you need to face, nonetheless, lie within these inquiries: What are you prepared to give up? What are you prepared to tolerate? What are you prepared to oppose? What are you prepared to do to achieve that transformative outcome?

I discovered that fitness is among the rare activities where privilege won't take you far without your full commitment to the effort.

Make your health important because someone you love or who loves you is always counting on you to stay alive.

Your health is sacred. There should be no excuse for neglecting its protection. You must be extravagant about it. You must lavish your time and energy on it. You must be willing to bleed or sweat for it if necessary, ache for it when applicable, and continue investing in it without apology.

Excellent health does not necessitate that we begin flawlessly or with ease. It simply anticipates that we start with a feeling of dedication and consistency. To obtain the outcomes you want, you must put in effort, even when resources are limited. You need to do it regularly, even when you're not very fond of it.

Nothing great happens by chance or coincidence. It takes commitment. It takes keeping your mouth silent, your mind open, and your hands doing the talking.

Start where you are and with what you have. That's how you build anything great that lasts. Always choose progression over flawlessness. It is never about who runs the fastest or who works the hardest. What really counts is who ends up going the furthest. To progress further, you just need to remain consistent with what is effective for you.

Even if you can allocate only a few minutes each day for yourself, don't overlook its significance. A daily increase of one percent is more advantageous than remaining completely unchanged every day. Every tiny step we make strengthens us further; every little action we take aids our wellness, and each completed session boosts our self-esteem.

Advancing your health positively isn't merely about who exerts the most effort or who sprints the fastest; it's about who maintains the greatest consistency. Moving too quickly can lead to exhaustion and fatigue. We may be enthusiastic about the notion of boundless energy and endorse these ideas since they attract significant attention, yet we are not machines, and we shouldn't tire ourselves out consistently to achieve good health. This is especially true if you aren't a fitness influencer whose motivation relies on posting about fitness daily.

Don't lose hope when others describe your goal as an insane concept. Indeed, a good indicator that your goal is sufficiently ambitious is when it leads others to underestimate your capacity to accomplish it. Individuals are constrained by their self-awareness, not by your understanding of yourself. If you think you can achieve it, then take action to realise it! It is your responsibility to demonstrate your abilities by accomplishing your objective.

Keep this in mind today: every day that ends with hope is a victory. It's normal to feel frustrated with your advancement. It's fine to feel exhausted by the extent to which it tires you out. It's normal to feel frustrated by how fast time is moving and that not much is going your way. It's alright to consider much of what you need to tackle at the moment challenging and difficult to bear. Regardless of the cards you have in your hand at this moment, do not give up. Accepting mediocrity won't simplify things, but appearing and finishing your workout sessions will.

A great approach to handling the challenges of your fitness journey is to stop worrying about the duration required to achieve your goals and instead concentrate on the joy of moving away from your current state, which does not bring you happiness. Once you depart from your current location and reach your desired destination, the feelings of pain and discomfort experienced during the journey will fade from your memory.

If you solely engage in what pleases you, you will keep experiencing outcomes that you despise. Any form of growth, although it is personal and subjective, is not mainly about preference but instead about progress. You may not enjoy every aspect, but if it proves effective, it's probably your best route to success.

You cannot be unhappy with your current situation, feel content while being inactive, and anticipate any improvements. Every day, you need to rise, prioritise your intention above all, and envision the life you want, disregard the challenges ahead, and just pursue it. Winning is impossible without being involved. You need to have the bravery and trust in yourself to achieve great success. The greater the number of excuses you offer or the more you waver, the sooner you begin to fail. There can't be successes without taking chances.

Achieving fitness doesn't mean we need to do anything extraordinary or use any fancy gear. It's more affordable than the social world has made us think in this contemporary era. Health is highly sought after, and certain individuals in the fitness sector have exploited this trend. Consequently, it is a business concern for them instead of your level of fitness. For you, this is centred on fitness, so let your exercise and diet prioritise your personal health and well-being.

At times, you simply need to rise from your bed and take action. It's all about getting ahead of your thinking by just diving in before you engage in a compromising discussion about it. That's how you accomplish tasks, even when you're not in the mood.

I just woke up one day and decided that it was my turn and time to benefit from my effort, time, and energy. We can spend our whole lives giving away our natural resources or redirect a significant part of them toward our happiness. Life offers no refunds; when a day is gone, you can't reclaim it unless you've used it wisely today for benefits in the future.

I started seeing real health gains when I stopped being inconsistent with my workouts. Nonetheless, one lesson I gained is to maintain consistency in a healthy way, which signifies acting sensibly. Indeed, on paper, exercising every day of the week seems impressive, commendable, and almost superhuman, but what other health consequences might it entail? Initially, exercising daily at the same intensity felt like I was winning, but I was actually worsening my health. I came to understand that consistency isn't about going to the gym seven days a week or avoiding calories 24/7. Rather, it is about balance and efficiency, as opposed to a dependence on intensity or speed. It's about not giving up, instead of overworking yourself continuously until you feel completely exhausted physically, mentally, and emotionally. Being consistent isn't about spending your energy and time excessively but simply about spreading their cost-effectively and in an affordable way.

www.ingramcontent.com/pod-product-compliance
Lightning Source LLC
Chambersburg PA
CBHW071240020426
42333CB00015B/1555